Burn Fat Fast:
Ridiculously Effective Flab Busting Secrets Revealed

By

Marc McLean

©Copyright 2017

By Marc McLean – All rights reserved

Author's Legal Disclaimer

This book is solely for informational and educational purposes and is not medical advice. Please consult a medical or health professional before you begin any new exercise, nutrition or supplementation program, or if you have questions about your health.

The information in this book is not a prescription and does not make any claim about health improvements, or any difference to your health in its own right. There are many elements to good health.

Any use of the information within this book is at the reader's discretion and risk. The author cannot be held responsible for any loss, claim or damage arising out of the use, or misuse, of the suggestions made, the failure to take medical advice, or for any related material from third party sources. No part of this publication shall be reproduced, transmitted, or sold in any form without the prior written consent of the author.

All trademarks and registered trademarks appearing in this digital book are the property of their respective owners.

Table of Contents

Introduction 1

Part One: It's Not Just What You Eat… 5

Say Goodbye To That Damn, Stubborn, Annoying, Lingering Fat… 6

Introducing Intermittent Fasting 10

It's As Simple As Skipping Breakfast 13

Success Stories 16

Learning From The Experts 19

Part Two: Exercise Like A Boss 22

Lift Weights (Heavy Only Please) 23

How Often - And How Long - Should You Be Training For? 27

The Fat Loss Fast Lane 29

Eight Reasons Why You Should Be Sprinting 31

Rapid Steps To Sprint Success 37

Tabata Training 42

Part Three: No Nonsense Nutrition 45

Sugar Ain't So Sweet 46

Eating Clean Made Simple 49

Why Energy Drinks Are To Be Avoided 54

Keeping Your Calories In Check 59

Delay Your Post-Workout Shake 62

One Positive Habit Per Week 64

Part Four: Fat Burning Hacks 69

Training In The Morning On An Empty Stomach ... 70

Supercharge Your Workouts With Black Coffee 73

Give Green Tea The Green Light 77

The Magic Of Lemon Water 79

Conclusion 84

About The Author 90

Introduction

Burning bodyfat is one of the easiest things in the world to do…

Yes easy. Yet so many people make such hard work of it. Sweating through boring exercise sessions that they don't really enjoy. Making themselves miserable eating salads, low fat foods and struggling like hell resisting their favourite treats.

Then they step on the scales a few weeks later, see that they've barely lost a single pound, and then lose the plot. Frustration reaches boiling point and there's only one thing for it…

Order a Chinese takeaway, get that half eaten tub of ice cream out the freezer, head to the shop and buy 17 bars of chocolate.

Does any of this sound even slightly familiar to you? Most of us who are less than happy with the shape we're in end up on the same merry-go-round of training/dieting > getting pissed off at the lack of results > going on a junk food bender > ending up back at square one.

It doesn't have to be that way. This book is your saviour! Follow the advice in the following chapters and you'll be able to turn your body into a fat burning machine.

I'll say it again: burning fat and staying lean is actually easy. It's just that most men and women go the wrong way about it.

Exercising ineffectively. Trying to eat healthily but doing so in an unhealthy way by following fad diets, or nutrition plans that are just way too complicated. The usual end result is failure simply because it's too difficult to maintain in the long run.

Fact is: nutrition accounts for about 70% of your success when it comes to achieving your health and fitness goals. If you're following an extreme diet or super strict nutrition plan then it's going to end in disaster as some point. Sure, you might get some results at first but you'll eventually lose willpower (and possibly the will to live!) and will inevitably return to old habits and pile the weight back on again.

What this book preaches is not only healthy eating, but a *healthy way of eating* that is sensible, do-able and manageable. You won't wanna punch me in the face after a week of following my nutritional advice. Notice that I say nutritional advice; we don't do 'diets' around here. Diets are unnatural, unnecessary and the results they bring are usually only temporary.

Here's more good news: you'll still be able to eat your favourite foods (without going mental) and lose weight. Everything in moderation is acceptable because the strategies in this book will elevate your metabolism levels (which equals fat burned) and will also force your body to use up its fat stores (…yes, even more fat incinerated).

How To Burn Fat Fast is split into four sections covering meal timing, exercise, nutrition, and fat burning hacks. These are the key areas for your success and each of them has ultra effective strategies that have a proven track record for creating fine, lean human specimens!

Combine all of the strategies included in these chapters and it's virtually impossible not to lose weight fast. If you do all of the above consistently, I'm pretty confident you'll be amazed at your body transformation. It doesn't matter how many times you've failed in the past, how overweight you are, or whether you're a man or woman. These tactics will blitz your bodyfat. I've witnessed it time and again with personal training clients, and friends and family who hound me for training/nutritional advice to lose fat.

The best part? It's not as hard as you think. You can potentially see a quick shift in your weight within the first week simply by following the ultra effective meal timing advice in chapter one. It might take a bit longer, along with combining the exercise strategies in part two, and the fat burning hacks in part four.

This is simply because we're all different. Our bodies are all various shapes and sizes, we have different metabolic rates, some readers are younger and more physically able than others. These factors all play a part in how quickly your bodyfat levels drop and your body shape changes. But you CAN do it.

Of course, it takes action, commitment and consistency from you too. You're more than capable of managing everything I describe in this book…and becoming a leaner, healthier, better version of yourself!

Part One

It's Not Just What You Eat...

Say Goodbye To That Damn, Stubborn, Annoying, Lingering Fat…

I had no idea so many guys struggled shifting the flab from their bellies. No clue that countless women think they are fat. And I didn't realise that so many people were doing so many ineffective things to try and get in shape.

People always tell me, "it's easy for you to say, you've always been slim." True - the main reason I kick-started my obsession with weight training and health and fitness in general back in 1998 was because I was so skinny. I hated being built like a rake and this created personal body image issues that most overweight people have too.

So I'm afraid I simply haven't got an amazing personal success story of how I went from fatboy to slimshady in a matter of weeks. Or shocking before and after pictures to prove it. Instead, I'll share several stories of clients, friends and family who have achieved just that - by following my training, nutrition and lifestyle advice. That very same advice is included in this book so you can finally hit your own health and fitness goals, and be proud of the new you.

When I set up my online personal training business last year I ran a Facebook advert to get clients for my men's body transformation programme. I asked people to fill in a questionnaire about their fitness goals and was expecting guys to be asking me to show them "how to build bigger biceps", "gain muscle mass", or simply learn how to create bigger, stronger bodies.

The responses I got surprised me. Out of nearly 50 guys from around the UK, more than half said their main goal was to lose weight or get rid of their belly fat. Below are some of their comments (I've not included their full names or locations because I don't have their permission).

David: "While I've achieved a slimmer physique, there is still some flab around my waist and I cannot develop visible muscle or a six pack."

Colin: "I want to bring my stomach in and lose weight overall."

Sid: "I'd like to lose weight for my high cholesterol, aswell as to be able to wear clothes I've not been able to wear for a while."

Spencer: "The biggest challenge is getting rid of the fat on my body. I can never lose it properly no matter what I try. I lose a bit then plateau and cannot break through to lose the gut where the majority of fat seems to sit."

Richard: "My problem is shedding fat around the love handles. It is going gradually but it just takes ages!"

Can you relate to any of these problems? If you're a woman it may be that you're desperate to lose weight from your hips, thighs or butt as these are lower body regions where females naturally store more bodyfat. For guys, the problem areas are primarily the upper body and belly.

I also asked the guys about their current weekly training regime and what their diet was like. You'd think that a chunk of them just didn't exercise enough but some of these guys were exercising 4 or 5 days per week, and their diets didn't seem too unhealthy (based on what they told me).

Why then were they all facing the same stumbling blocks? Why could they just not shift that damn, stubborn, annoying, lingering fat?

Firstly, how many days you train or how long you exercise for is not quite as important. The type of exercise - and the intensity of it - is what separates the mediocre results from the marvellous.

Secondly, these people had no clue about the calories they were taking in and expending each day. Calories are important; and if the input is more than the output consistently then you're inevitably going to put on weight. Don't worry, I'm not expecting you to start counting calories every time you eat - that would just be ridiculous. However, it's important you have a rough idea of your daily calorie intake and I'm going to share with you a tactic that makes this so easy to track.

Thirdly, none of these guys were implementing the full range of fat burning hacks that I reveal in Part Four.

And finally, not one of them had employed - or even heard of - what I consider the single most effective tactic for stripping bodyfat (while maintaining lean muscle). This is the number one piece of advice I give to men and women looking to burn fat and develop a leaner body. Some of my clients have seen some outstanding results with it. It's backed by solid science, it has numerous other health benefits, and it's much easier to implement than hopping about from one crazy fad diet to another.

I'm talking about…intermittent fasting.

Introducing Intermittent Fasting

What was your first reaction when you read "intermittent fasting" on the previous page?

Did the voice in your head say something like: "Fuck this, I'm not fasting…I'm not really into starving!"

Unless you've already heard about intermittent fasting and are clued-up on how it works, then that's the kind of response I get from most people when I first mention those words. They might not say it, but I can see from the reaction on their faces that the word "fasting" has put the fear into them.

I'm going to give a simple explanation about how it works, how I first came across it five or six years ago, and I'll also serve up a few stories of personal training clients and friends who've experienced amazing results with intermittent fasting.

First, let's get a few things straight.

Intermittent fasting is NOT:

- Some sort of diet plan, it simply involves adjusting the time you eat your meals.

- Hard to stick with, in fact it's much easier than following any fad diet.

- Dangerous or unhealthy in any way, in fact it has numerous health benefits.

- Reliant on willpower, it's just a case of your body adjusting to a new eating schedule.

Intermittent fasting IS:

- An effective way of burning fat without going on a super restrictive diet.

- A more natural way of eating which harks back to the 'hunter gatherer' days of our ancestors.

- Beneficial for your digestive system as gives it a rest from breaking down large volumes of food often.

- Backed by science as an effective way of regenerating your cells and boosting your immune system.

How Intermittent Fasting Works

So what is intermittent fasting? It means having an extended break between your meals in order to trigger a natural fat burning response in your body. Our body builds up glycogen stores from the food we eat and this is our main source of energy for our activities and to get through the day.

When we go for long breaks without food our glycogen bank run out - and our body is forced to turn to bodyfat for energy.

How long is that break without food? Generally a period of 14-18 hours. Once you get beyond the 14 hour mark of no food supply, the body will eat into fat stores for energy. As you get nearer the 18 hour mark, more and more coal is being added to your body's fat burning fire.

I know what you're thinking…"how the hell am I going to last without food for 14 hours or more?" That may sound like torture at first, but it's easier than you think because this period also takes into account your sleeping hours.

When we're sleeping we're effectively fasting for 8 hours, or however long you're snoozing. All we have to do next is extend that by another six hours and we're in the fat burning zone.

It's As Simple As Skipping Breakfast

You can achieve your intermittent fasting goal simply by skipping breakfast. All you have to do is ensure there's at least a 14 hour gap between your last meal in the evening and your first meal the following day.

It's flexible and here's how it can play out easily in various ways…

Scenario 1: You finish eating dinner with the family at 8pm, go to bed a few hours later, and then head to work without eating breakfast. But you're a clever dude and have packed some food on-the-go in your bag and whip them out in the office at 11am. So, 8pm-11am is a break of 15 hours - job done!

Scenario 2: You get in from work late and dinner has basically become supper as you're now finishing it at 9.30pm. No sweat because you skip breakfast the following day and don't eat lunch until 12noon. That's an intermittent fasting period of 14.5 hours - job done!

Scenario 3: It's 10am and you're feeling really hungry. You remember that the last time you ate yesterday was around 6pm…so that means there's already a 16 hour intermittent fasting period. You're good to go.

I think you get the picture. The times you eat can be flexible and can fit around your life. It's basically just a case of making sure there's a gap of at least 14 hours between your last meal your first meal today and your last meal yesterday.

You may still not be 100% sold on the idea, thinking it's going to be too difficult to maintain. Trust me, it's easier than you think - and definitely much easier than following extreme diets where various foods are completely banned.

Intermittent fasting simply focuses on the *timing* of your meals, rather than the *foods included* in your meals. No foods are banned and it certainly gives you a bit more freedom when it comes to your daily food choices. That being said, I don't recommend eating a multi-pack of Mars bars the minute you exceed the 14 hour mark of your fast. That's not exactly gonna work.

I'll go into nutrition and the types of foods you should be eating - and avoiding - in Part Three. I'm just trying to make the point that intermittent fasting is a completely new approach to losing weight and keeping it off.

If you've tried all sorts of diets to burn fat and got nowhere, this single tactic might well be the answer to your prayers. I say that confidently because I've seen it work wonders with clients who struggled big time with their weight.

While I've always been a naturally slimmer guy who finds it hard to gain weight, I also follow intermittent fasting because it keeps my bodyfat levels low effortlessly. I eat a clean diet Monday-Friday and train hard 3-4 days per week, but at the weekend I eat junk food that would otherwise result in a flabby belly. It never happens - because intermittent fasting (and my heavy weight training regime) compensates and keeps me in great shape.

Success Stories

I got a Facebook private message from Colin McIntyre - a guy I hadn't heard from in years - in November 2016. He wrote: "Are you still doing personal training? I'd really like you to help me get into shape?"

Here's my disclaimer upfront - Colin is my cousin, so he's obviously going to say nothing but good things about the help I gave him! But I'm relaying his story here because I think it's one that many readers will be able to relate to.

Colin's a married dad-of-two, who works long hours, and admitted that maintaining a healthy diet was always his biggest struggle. He'd reached his heaviest ever weight and was desperate to get rid of his overhanging belly.

First, we swapped his running for lifting heavy weights. Next, he was expecting a strict, rigid meal plan from me. That's not exactly how it worked out.

Rather than ban all sorts of foods and insist that Colin lives on chicken and steamed broccoli most of the week, I simply instructed him to skip breakfast every day and following some foundational nutritional advice (as described later in Part Three).

Here's what happened…

"For years I used to go out running for miles to try and get in decent shape," said Colin. "It was usually the same route, it was usually boring as hell, and I was lucky if I lost one, maybe two pounds.

"I'd just get fed up after 2-3 weeks and go back to eating junk food again. After joining Marc's programme and doing the intermittent fasting I dropped 15lbs in the first month alone.

"Everyone could see the difference in me. My boss had been off work for 6 weeks and when he came back the first thing he said to me was, 'man, you've lost some weight!'

"I went through the Christmas and New Year period afterwards expecting to gain some weight again but it stayed at the same level. I was really surprised at that."

Intermittent fasting was undoubtedly a big factor in Colin's success as diet was the big problem area for him, but combining this with my specific weight training programme supercharged his results. (We move onto the brilliant fat-burning benefits of lifting weights in Part Two).

Chris Hannan signed up to my body transformation programme in March this year because he had a holiday coming up. He'd also piled on the weight and wanted to burn fat fast before hitting the beach.

"My holiday is in a fortnight…do you think I can lose some weight by then?", he said.

He didn't exactly give me much time to work a miracle, but I was confident intermittent fasting would deliver surprising results. Chris was simply advised to skip breakfast, cut his calories slightly, lift weights three times per week, and limit sugar/junk foods.

The result? He lost 10lbs in 10 days, more than he expected before his holiday. As I've just mentioned, there were several changes to Chris' lifestyle in terms of nutrition and training, but intermittent fasting was undoubtedly the most effective element.

Learning From The Experts

Considering how effective it is and how easy it is to follow, I'm surprised the intermittent fasting phenomenon isn't more widespread. The word is slowly getting out there and I've recently spoken to a few gym instructors who have educated themselves on its benefits and are passing the message on.

I first came across the fasting approach about five or six years ago after buying the book 'The Warrior Die't by Ori Hofmekler. Author of several health and fitness/sports nutrition books and founder of Defense Nutrition, Ori's knowledge of sports science and how the human body works is on a different planet.

The premise of The Warrior Diet is that we fast during the day - and feast at night. He argues that this is how we as humans are biologically engineered to survive because in caveman days humans would often spend many hours during the day hunting for food, and then would eat their 'catch' by the fire at night.

Ori explains how this approach of fasting for a long period and feasting during a smaller window ramps up fat burning and helps create a leaner, more athletic body. Big name athletes who follow The Warrior Diet include former women's world UFC champion Ronda Rousey and kettlebell expert Pavel Tsatsouline.

Now aged 65, Ori is in better shape than most guys in their 20's.

That was my first introduction to the concept of intermittent fasting, and I was completely sold on it after reading the book 'Eat Stop Eat' by Brad Pilon. While researching the book, nutritional expert Brad reviewed hundreds of scientific papers and reviews into the effects of intermittent fasting.

There had been some claims by sceptics and critics that fasting for extended periods could cause metabolic damage or lead to health issues in the long term.

In the book, Brad writes: "Almost all of the scientific research I reviewed provided evidence in direct opposition to the misinformation found in diet books and on the internet. I found very convincing evidence that supports the use of short term fasting as an effective weight loss tool.

"This included research on the effect that fasting has on your memory and cognitive abilities, your metabolism and muscle, and the effect that fasting has on exercise and exercise performance."

How Long Should You Fast?

If you want to delve deeper into the workings of intermittent fasting, or the science behind it, then I'd highly recommend Brad's book Eat Stop Eat. He's the main man when it comes to this particular area and I've yet to read a better book on this single topic.

Are you ready to give it a go (and I highly recommend you do) but are not sure how long you should be fasting for? 14 hours, 15…18?

There's no one definitive answer because how quickly we burn fat depends on various factors including our age, activity level, metabolic rate etc. Fourteen hours is typically the minimum period before fat burning really begins to kick in, and for me personally the sweet spot is 14-16 hours.

For those who are very overweight or want to have the best chance of burning fat fastest, then I'd aim for 16-18 hours between your first meal of the day and last meal the previous day.

I've seen intermittent fasting work wonders. I'm certain it can do the same for you.

Part Two

Exercise Like A Boss

Lift Weights (Heavy Only Please)

I'm always banging on about lifting weights to anyone that'll listen…

My 93-year-old neighbour. The woman that served me in Aldi yesterday. Random folk I see looking bored to tears on the treadmill. That's because most people have got the wrong idea about weight training.

It's NOT all about building muscle…

It's not just for fitter, stronger, younger people…

Or guys wearing muscle vests and make loud grunting noises in the gym.

Weight training/strength training is highly effective for burning fat - much more so than standard cardio exercise. For some reason, many people still think that cardio is for fat loss and weight training is for muscle gain. Like it's that black and white.

I was speaking to a friend of a friend in the gym last week who doing bench presses, barbell biceps curls and a couple of other really effective weight training exercises. But then he cut his weights session short to head for the cardio machines.

He told me: "I'm enjoying lifting some weights and I'm feeling stronger but I'm doing 30 minutes of cardio next because I need to lose this flab around my belly. I just can't seem to shift it."

His split exercise approach - doing a half-hearted weights session and half-assed cardio workout - was clearly one of the main problems.

Same thing happened a few days later when I bumped into an old schoolmate in the gym. He was looking for advice to get in shape. I asked him what his main goals were and what he'd been doing up until now to try and achieve them.

He said: "I want to add more muscle up top, in my chest area, shoulders and arms. I've been doing weight training nearly every day the past two weeks.

"I'm not getting any younger and I've got a bit of a pot belly these days, so I'm also playing five-a-side football and doing sit-ups at home."

Another flawed approach for two reasons. One - he was lifting weights too frequently which will hamper results and lead to burnout in the long run. A better approach is to give the body roughly around 48 hours to recover if you're training properly with heavy weights at the right intensity.

Secondly, he'd also bought into the notion that cardio exercise and a ton of sit-ups will get rid of his bulging belly. Afraid not.

Weight Training Develops Lean Muscle AND Burns Bodyfat

The reality is that cardio burns some calories, can help you lose some fat (in an inefficient way), and it does zilch for muscle tone.

Meanwhile, weight training keeps calories burning long after you stop training. Studies have shown that heavy resistance training can keep metabolism levels elevated up to 24 hours after exercise. With standard cardio training this 'after-burn' period is much shorter. Weight training also sparks muscle development and remodelling through a process called hypertrophy (aka muscle tissue growth). How do you reach hypertrophy effectively? By lifting heavy weights and pushing yourself hard in the gym.

I'm a huge fan of 'compound exercises' and these are the moves that make up the majority of my workouts and the training plans of my online PT clients. I'm talking about the big moves that have been proven and delivered awesome results since some strong dude in a cave invented weight training.

The compound moves include: squats, deadlifts, chin-ups, bent over row, upright row…and a few more. I cover all the top compound weight training exercises, muscle isolation exercises, and reveal my top training strategies in the book 'Strength Training Program 101: Build Muscle & Burn Fat…In Less Than 3 Hours Per Week'. It's available via Amazon and also features a bonus exercise demo guide to help readers master every move.

The reason compounds work so well is that they work various muscle groups at once and trigger the release of more anabolic hormones in the body. This basically means more muscle, less fat. We'll talk more about stimulating that anabolic response and the role of individual hormones in the body in the next chapter.

How Often - And How Long - Should You Be Training For?

How pissed off are you with your current body shape? How much do you want rid of the belly? How frustrating is it when you look in the mirror after weeks of training and dieting and see zero changes?

For many people the desperate need for change fires up their motivation levels to the extent where they're willing to train 5,6,7 days per week. They'll get up at stupid o'clock to do a fitness class before work. They'll drag themselves to the gym even when they're not feeling it after a long day.

Of course, that's the right attitude. You do have to work hard, do it consistently, and keep your nutrition on point to get the results you really want. But what if I told you that exercising barely three hours per week is enough to burn bodyfat, get lean and transform your bodyshape?

That's exactly what I'm telling you - if you train in the right manner. I'm sure you've already got the message that I'm not a fan of cardio. Weight training is the way because it does a 3 for 1 job: builds muscle, strips bodyfat and sculpts a leaner, more athletic physique overall. (There are countless other benefits as well such as improved heart health, stronger bones, better posture…these are all covered in my Strength Training Program 101 book).

Training in the right manner means lifting heavy weights with a lower amount of reps, and continually increasing the resistance on your muscles to trigger hypertrophy. The strain on your muscles will/should always leave you feeling sore as a result over the next 24-48 hours (sometimes longer for beginners), which means you must give your body sufficient rest to recover.

That's why I always recommend training **<u>one day on, one day off</u>** when it comes to lifting weights. (i.e. Monday, Wednesday, Friday). By focusing on various compound exercises you work many different muscle groups and ensure an all-over body workout more efficiently too - meaning your gym session can easily be finished in 45-60 mins. The only time I'm in the gym longer than an hour is if I'm wasting time talking to people or watching music videos of Rihanna on the TV. Or Beyonce. Or Taylor Swift.

Want a highly effective way to burn bodyfat - and keep it burning long after you step out of the gym? Then it's time to hit the weights section.

The Fat Loss Fast Lane

Did you ever watch the Olympics when you were a kid? Did it ever leave you a bit confused?

That's what happened with me. I loved the 100m sprint. It was fast, exciting and all of the guys competing were my vision of what a perfect athlete should look like. They always had strong powerful legs, broad shoulders, a rounded chest, bulging biceps, and perfect muscle definition - all with hardly a trace of bodyfat. To round it all off they were as quick as lightning.

Then I'd watch the 10,000m…and the runners were built like toothpicks. It looked likethey needed a meal more than any medal.

What was going on? Both groups of athletes were runners – but they had completely different physiques. I just couldn't get my head round it.

Turns out that these types of running trigger a different physiological response in the body. Long distance running is catabolic (aka breaks down muscle tissue) while sprinting is anabolic (builds muscle tissue).

The main reason for this is that the high intensity - all-out - power surge - of sprints in short bursts absolutely supercharges the body's production of growth hormone. One of the primary anabolic hormones, growth hormone is one of the key players in muscle growth and development.

Here's the big bonus: **growth hormone also triggers lipolysis (fat breakdown) and also causes fatty acids to be utilised by the body**. So it's essentially a two-for-one with sprint training - develop lean muscle while stripping fat at the same time.

Want to burn fat fast? Then it's time to start running fast. I mean flat out. Till you feel like your heart is going to burst through your chest.

On your marks. Get set…

Eight Reasons Why You Should Be Sprinting

Go out for a jog and you'll raise your heart rate, increase your metabolic rate, burns some calories, and then your body's systems will return back to normal fairly shortly afterwards.

Running at full speed - like you're being chased by an axe murderer - for just 10-15 seconds is on a whole other level. As I mentioned in the previous chapter, there's something special about sprinting that sparks a supercharged response in the endocrine system. It floods your body with muscle building, fat burning growth hormone, and sparks a surge of other anabolic hormones too.

Yet again, just like weight training, this means fat loss and muscle development at the same time. Now *that's* why Olympic sprinters - the men and the women - have bodies like Greek Gods. I don't think I've seen a female 100m sprint athlete without awesome abs.

Best of all: a single sprints training session can be done in as little as 15-20 mins. Below I list eight great reasons why you – and every fit and able person – should be sprinting.

#1 It can more than QUADRUPLE growth hormone production

Growth hormone is known for stimulating growth, cell regeneration and reproduction. As well as those fat burning benefits I've just described, growth hormone also plays various other roles in the body including enhancing immune system function.

So you can clearly see why doing anything that increases your levels of growth hormone is a good move when it comes to burning fat and improving your overall body shape.

Sprinting doesn't just give growth hormone a little boost – it supercharges it. A study published in The Journal of Sports Sciences in June 2002 showed that sprinting more than **quadrupled** growth hormone production.

Nine men completed two sprints – one for six seconds and another for 30 seconds – and had blood samples taken afterwards. Growth hormone levels were 450% higher after the 30 secs sprint compared to the short six second burst. These levels also stayed elevated for 90-120 minutes afterwards. Pretty amazing stuff!

#2 It kickstarts the other anabolic hormones too…

Sprinting may well turn you into an anabolic muscle growing, fat burning machine…because it also raises levels of the other primary anabolic hormones, testosterone and IGF1.

This was shown in another study published in The Journal of Strength And Conditioning Research in August 2011. The research involved 12 young men and highlighted that levels of testosterone and IGF1, along with growth hormone, were all elevated after various sprints involving distances of 100m-400m.

#3 It torches fat

Sprinting is like adding a heap of coal to your fat burning fire because it revs up your metabolism and keeps stripping fat long after your workout.

This form of training **increased fat oxidation by 75%**, according to research from February 2013. Researchers had 10 healthy men, aged 21-27, perform four 30 second bouts of cycle sprints, followed by almost five minutes of rest.

Aswell as the massive increase in fat oxidation, blood pressure levels were also shown to be reduced afterwards.

#4 It's a super efficient way to train

Your sprinting session should be finished in 15-20 mins. That's it. It simply involves intense bursts of speed over short distances, followed by quick breathers. Therefore it's a super efficient and ultra effective way to train.

Do it in the morning – on an empty stomach – for the best effect. In the previous study I mentioned above where the guys increased fat oxidation by 75%, they had all fasted overnight.

The significance of this is that your body's glycogen stores are lower after a period of fasting. If you haven't eaten since the previous evening when you sprint your body will turn to fatty acids for fuel…which equals an even better fat burn.

#5 It's a shortcut to a six-pack

The number one reason you've not got a six pack yet is not because you're not doing enough crunches. It's not because you had too much pasta on Tuesday night…

It's because your bodyfat levels are not low enough.

The abdominal muscles are there – but to get them on show you gotta remove the layer of fat that's camouflaging them. We've already seen how sprinting takes fat burning to new levels, while preserving and developing muscle mass. The exercise itself, thrusting your legs and arms forward powerfully at speed, also forces the abdominal muscles to work hard. I'd take 10 sprints over 1000 crunches any day.

#6 It improves heart health

Regular exercise is recommended for people with high blood pressure, and it appears that high intensity training is more effective than moderate exercise for improving the situation.

Comparing 30 minutes of moderate exercise to several bouts of high intensity (HIT) exercise, lasting 1-4 minutes, researchers concluded that HIT is "superior to CMT (continuous moderate training) for improving cardiorespiratory fitness".

Their findings published in the American Journal of Cardiovascular Disease in 2012 also showed that intense exercise was shown to have positive effects on arterial stiffness and insulin sensitivity.

#7 It strengthens the mind

Getting through a sprint session is tough, I won't lie. If it's your first time you'll feel like your heart is thumping, your mouth will be wide open trying to take in every tiny air particle, you'll think there's barely a drip of fuel left in the tank…

But that's the way it should be – and that's what will deliver all the other benefits ts listed above. Another big reason for sprinting is that it'll undoubtedly make you stronger mentally.

You've got to sprint so hard to the point where you think your body has nothing left to give. It's by pushing through and overcoming that mental battle that it'll strengthen your mind.

#8 It's a mood booster

We all know about the release of endorphins – feel good chemicals – that are stimulated by exercise, but this is heightened when you push yourself to the limit in this intense form of training. Especially when sprinting outside on a nice sunny morning.

My favourite time of year is spring and I love breathing in the fresh air with the sun shining on my sweaty face after an intense all-out sprint session. It sets you up for a positive day – I never have a bad day on a sprint day.

Different Types of Sprint Training

If you're still not convinced on sprinting then I'll eat my own stinking sweatyshoe after my sprint session tomorrow morning! Now we've discussed the main awesome benefits of sprint training, let's look at the three main options you have to get started.

- Standard sprints – on a flat surface, road or grass.
- Hill sprints – an incline will turn the intensity up a notch.
- Cycle sprints – all out pedalling with rest periods.

So let's just get this straight. Sprints supercharge growth hormone, get the body in an anabolic state to develop lean muscle mass, fire up fat burning, improve the health of your ticker, sculpt your six pack, strengthen the mind, make you feel amazing afterwards…and your workout is done in 15-20 minutes.

Have you pulled your running shoes on yet…?

Rapid Steps To Sprint Success

If you're ready to start sprinting then you had better get ready for some awesome results. But don't be thinking those results come easy. My friend introduced me to hill sprint training around 2011 – at a time when I thought I was in half decent shape and generally quite fit. An all-out sprint to the top of the hill, walk back down again, and repeat. What could be so hard about that?

The first sprint was pretty tough, I'd say 7/10. Reaching the top of the hill for my second one I was wheezing like an asthmatic, chest-infected chain-smoker. By the third I was gassed out – and thought I needed gas and air! That day I was planning on 10 hill sprints. I managed six.

The hill kicked my ass and showed me I wasn't nearly as fit as I thought I was. But...I was absolutely buzzing afterwards for still pushing through when I was really struggling after that third sprint.

I stuck at it, doing two sprint sessions per week outside on a hill near my house. My fitness improved quickly and I gradually increased the number of sprints and extended the distance as I progressed. Within a month the six pack abs I hadn't seen since I was about 18 were back. To be honest, my stomach was always flat and I could *feel* abdominal muscles – but up until that point you couldn't see them because they were well hidden by a layer of fat. Sprints stripped that fat away when all the other exercises I tried didn't.

You can benefit from the immense fat burn, while preserving and developing muscle as explained in the previous chapter. Here's how to get started and should progress as you gradually improve your sprinting performance and overall fitness.

ROOKIE (just starting out...)

Distance: 50-60 yards.

Sprints: 5-6.

>>> Head to your local park, or somewhere else outside, and locate a stretch of flat ground that's not very busy with people. (You want to be able to do your sprints uninterrupted without trying to swerve round people). >>> Choose a starting point and set a marker around 50-60 yards away, i.e. a park bench or street light. >>> Warm up for five minutes by jogging on the spot, doing star jumps, squats...and anything else that makes you feel slightly stupid outside! Seriously, the warm-up is important so also add-in various stretches for your legs and upper body too before you get started. >>> On your marks...sprint as fast as you possibly can to your marker point. As soon as you reach it walk back towards where you started, breathing in deep through

your nose to get plenty of oxygen back in your lungs. >>> Once you get to the starting point, turn and set off again, running as fast as you can. >>> Repeat for 5-6 sprints.

INTERMEDIATE (have done sprints before, ready for more action...)

Distance: 100 yards.

Sprints: 8-9.

>>> Go to your local park, or somewhere else outside, and find a clear stretch of flat ground – or a spot with a slight incline. >>> Choose a starting spot and set a marker around 100 yards away. >>> Always make sure you warm up properly for five minutes before you begin. >>> Then, like above, sprint at maximum effort till you reach your marker and then walk back to the beginning. >>> Rinse and repeat for 8-9 sprints.

ADVANCED (Mr Bolt needs a 1 second head start on you...)

Distance: 120-150 yards.

Sprints: 10-12.

>>> Find a hill, or road with an incline (but not too steep...or else your calves will be on fire for the rest of the month). >>> Choose a starting point and set a marker further away this time, around 120-150 yards. >>> As ever, ensure you warm up well with stretches, jogging on the spot etc. >>> Using the same simple sprint/rest protocol, do this until you complete between 10 and 12 full sprints at maximum effort. Below I share with you my 11 point checklist to make sure you don't trip yourself up with schoolboy errors and instead get the most out of your sprint sessions.

Sprinter's Checklist

1. Set your alarm. Get up early to do your hill sprints before breakfast to maximise the fat burn.

2. Wear decent training shoes. Nice light ones.

3. Load music on to your iPhone...or whatever music player you use. You're gonna need good tunes to get you through to the end.

4. Wear tracksuit bottoms with a zip pocket...to keep your phone/music player in. I cracked the screen on my last iPhone after it fell out of my pocket when I was going at full-speed. It's also a pain in the ass running while holding your phone in your hand.

5. Take some handkerchiefs/toilet roll. Your nose will likely be dripping.

6. Don't forget to warm-up. Do a light jog and also take around 5 minutes doing some leg and arm stretches, running on the spot, bodyweight squats etc.

7. Take a bottle of water. You'll definitely be needing some h2o pronto afterwards.

8. Don't time yourself. It's a hassle and you're too busy fumbling around trying to start and stop the timer that you don't launch yourself off or finish properly. Just aim to go flat out from start to finish.

9. Set yourself a target number of sprints and stick to it. At least 5 as a rookie - and eventually work your way up to 12.

10. Don't give up. It's gonna be tough, no doubt about it but you gotta keep going.

11. Enjoy it. It may be tough physically and mentally just getting through the intense session but the buzz afterwards is amazing. The feel good endorphins will be bursting out your ears and it'll totally set you up for a great day.

Tabata Training

"Don't sit down, keep moving around…"

I can still hear the Australian voice repeating those words through the gym music system. I was a sweating, shaking, quivering mess and was wondering where the hell I was going to find the energy to get through the rest of the workout. I seriously thought I might spew - and that's exactly why there was always a sick bucket in the room during these intense sessions. My mate Alan Nisbet had plenty of fun filling that with his half-digested dinner on several occasions.

This was around 12 years ago and the first time I'd been introduced to 'Tabata' training…or done any proper high intensity interval training (HIIT) really. It was at the D-Unit Sports Combat Hub where I live in Alexandria, Scotland, and this special form of training was initially used to get the club's group of mixed martial arts stars in peak condition for their upcoming fights.

It involved doing various exercise drills at full capacity with very limited rest for almost an hour. It was punishing and, while I always thought I was fit as fuck, this proved I never really had the stamina I thought I had. The classes were then opened up to the local community and are still a big hit with hundreds of people every week at the D-Unit.

While I barely survived and just managed to hold in my puke, I loved how the Tabata system worked and was impressed after researching the science behind it. So much so that I now often apply it to the end of my weight training sessions, which I'll talk about later in this chapter.

Tabata training essentially involves 20 secs of exercise at maximum effort, followed by 10 secs rest, repeated for eight rounds. This short, sharp burst of training (just like sprints) is over very quickly…but the high level of intensity has the effect of elevating metabolism, and increasing the fat burn for up to 12 hours afterwards.

Now you're probably thinking, "I thought he said he didn't like cardio." I know, I'm a two-faced fucker. But I don't really class Tabata training or sprint training as cardio because they create such a unique physiological response in the body. Devised by Japanese scientist Dr Izumi Tabata, this professor did trials with Olympians and his findings were that Tabata training was more effective than other forms of HIIT for improving aerobic and anaerobic fitness.

Applying Tabata Training To Your Workouts

I like to throw in a Tabata style short session at the end of my weight training workouts to ramp up fat burning. This always involves lighter weights because you're pushing yourself harder for an extended period with minimal rest, rather than having a decent break in between three weightlifting sets.

For example, I might do squats with a 20kg weight bag resting on my shoulders, or bench press with a light weight. Twenty seconds work, 10 seconds rest, for the duration of the eight rounds.

I call it the workout 'finisher' and it definitely enhances the fat burning effect of your weights workout. There are plenty of free Tabata timer apps on the iTunes and Android stores that you can download to your phone for your workouts.

Personally, I'd recommend buying the 'Tabata Pro' timer app for £2.99. It's a cool, easy to use system, and also allows you to play your music at the same time (which can be a major help to get through a punishing Tabata round at the end of your workout).

Part Three

No Nonsense Nutrition

Sugar Ain't So Sweet

"Marc, what foods should I be cutting out to lose weight?"

"I don't really have a clue about a healthy diet. What should I be avoiding?"

"I've been eating low fat foods, but I've still not been losing any fat."

These are common questions I get from people via my weight training website, from friends, and even from my mum. But she still won't listen when I tell her to step away from the cakes. While intermittent fasting is always my number #1 piece of advice for anyone looking to burn bodyfat, making better food choices is obviously going to have a positive impact too. Stating the obvious with that one, but there's still a big misconception that eating high fat foods are what's making people fat.

Fat ain't the problem. <u>Sugar</u> is.

Consistently consume excessive amounts of sugar and it literally converts to bodyfat. Here's how it works…

Whenever we fill our bodies with too much fuel - which is very easy with high sugar foods - there's a glucose overload and the liver runs out of storage capacity. The excess sugar is converted into fatty acids and is then returned to the bloodstream. This is then stored as bodyfat in your belly, hips, chest and other areas you don't want it.

Too much sugar intake also results in insulin issues. Insulin is a key hormone in the body, and is released in high amounts whenever you eat or drink a "simple" carbohydrate, which includes the likes of white bread, white rice, baked white potato, bagels, croissants, cornflakes, cake, sugary drinks, beer, and anything that has high fructose corn syrup on the nutritional label.

When insulin levels are spiked the body's fat burning process is shut down so that the sugar that's just been consumed can be used for energy straight away. Sugar is shuttled into your muscles but, as soon as the muscle energy stores are full, the excess sugars are converted and stored as bodyfat.

So you can see that while it may taste oh so good at the time, sugar ain't so sweet for our bodyshape. It's also bad, very bad, for our health.

Cancer, heart disease, diabetes, metabolic syndrome and various other diseases have been strongly linked with over-consumption of refined sugar. Researchers at the University of California commented in the journal Nature that refined sugar contributes to around 35 million deaths around the world.

How Much Is Too Much?

The American Heart Association recommends that 37.5 grams (around 6 or 7 teaspoons) of added sugar is the daily limit for men, while 25g (around 5 teaspoons) is enough for women. To avoid going over the limit, ditching fizzy drinks and eating cakes and too much chocolate is wise move. And check the sugar content listed on nutritional labels on your food and drink.

Also, sugar is not always listed as sugar. Look out for the names of its man-made dodgy cousins including high fructose corn syrup, dried cane syrup and brown rice syrup. If there are several of them in the one food item then I'd steer clear.

Eating Clean Made Simple

Good nutrition accounts for about 70% of your fitness success, according to health experts.

Problem is, sticking to a healthy diet is where most of us struggle, right? If you're reading this now I'm guessing you've probably tried various diets or followed a nutrition plan devised by a PT in an attempt to get rid of excess bodyfat.

How did you find it? Was the food bland and boring? Was there too much meal prepping involved? Was it making you miserable trying to stick with it?

Fact is: if the 'diet' you're following is hard to maintain, not enjoyable, and feels like a strict military exercise then you're inevitably going to quit. That's the main reasons I take a different approach with personal training clients - and in my own life.

It's pointless me acting like a food Nazi, saying, "don't eat this…stay away from that…blah blah." Life's too short to put ourselves on ridiculous food bans. Everything in moderation is the way to go if it prevents us from quitting and eating a full tub of ice cream on a Wednesday night.

Four basic rules I stick by are:

- Eat clean Monday-Friday…and live a little at the weekend.

- Include plenty of whole foods in your diet (the stuff that grows in the ground and on trees).

- Cook fresh as much as possible.

- Limit sugar and processed foods (i.e. ready meals, sweets etc).

Enjoy your usual Chinese takeaway meal - but save it for the weekend. Have a little chocolate - just make sure it's not a king size bar. You get the idea.

If you follow those four basic rules, and combine them with intermittent fasting and regular exercise, you can't go wrong. You'll still be burning fat while not subjecting yourself to an extreme diet or unhealthy ways of eating that will only result in failure eventually.

My book 'Strength Training Nutrition 101: Build Muscle & Burn Fat Easily…A Healthy Way Of Eating You Can Actually Maintain' goes into much more detail on this. It also lists my top food sources for protein, carbohydrates and fat, guidelines on how much of these macronutrients you should be taking in based on your body type, and more.

While my approach is not to be the food police, I've still pulled together a list of foods that it's advisable to **avoid** as much as possible if you want to successfully burn fat and get leaner.

#1 Fizzy drinks

Cola, Pepsi, 7-Up…all these sugar-laden fizzy drinks are bad news for your waistline and your health. I already covered the dangers of too much sugar in the last chapter and how it converts to fat in the body. Downing fizzy drinks is like shuttling spoonful after spoonful of sugar into your mouth. Swap it for water, or diluting juice.

#2 White bread

White bread is not good for you. It lacks the fibre and several other nutrients that whole grain bread provides. Adding to the problem is the fact that white bread is not naturally white - the flour is chemically bleached to give it that colour. Yep, bleached. Best giving that a miss too.

#3 Cakes, sweets

I'm not sure I have to explain why here, but I will anyway. Cakes and sweets contain large amounts of sugar, often with hydrogenated fats which are damaging to your health. Remember, what I said about eating clean Monday-Friday and relaxing your diet a little at the weekend? Cakes and sweets should be left till the weekend.

#4 Beer/lager

Beer and lager will hamper your fat burning attempts for various reasons. Firstly, they contain more calories than most other alcoholic drinks. There are usually at least 200 calories in a pint of beer and I know guys who can easily drink 8-10 pints a night at the pub.

When we're heading home drunk we usually grab some sort of takeaway food, don't we? That's causing another problem because alcohol affects the body's ability to metabolise calories, causing them to be stored as fat rather than glycogen. When we're hungover the next day there's nothing healthy on the menu, only junk food will do! All in all, beer and lager are best avoided if you want to successfully burn fat.

#5 Margarine

My mum put margarine on my sandwiches all through primary school - it's no wonder I've turned out like this! Seriously, I don't know why this stuff even continues to sell. Margarine surged in popularity a couple of decades ago as an alternative to butter because there was the misconception that saturated fat was bad for us. Turns out it's the other way round. Margarine contains man-made trans-fats which are denatured and unhealthy to the body. Butter is the healthier, more natural and tastier choice.

#6 Vegetable oils

This follows the same kind of argument as above. Vegetable oils grew in popularity when health experts demonised saturated fats, believing they were bad for our health and caused heart disease. It is now widely accepted that saturated fat plays various important roles in the body including the manufacture of hormones and immune function. Vegetable oils meanwhile, such as sunflower, corn and canola oil, are less than healthy and are hard for the body to break down when heated.

Why Energy Drinks Are To Be Avoided

Every time I walk into the gym I can expect to count at least two or three drinks cans sitting in a corner on the floor.

There are countless brands of energy drinks being sold these days and there's a misconception that these will help you achieve your health and fitness goals quicker. I often see people downing them to get through their workouts, clearly thinking it'll give them a boost in performance and fire them up for a better workout. And a better workout equals more fat burnt, right?

In the case of energy drinks, no. In fact, it's completely defeating the purpose. You might feel wired and charged up due to the sky high levels of caffeine in these energy drinks, but some of them also contain up to **17 teaspoons of sugar!** This is more than DOUBLE the recommended amount of daily added sugar. As explained earlier, excess sugar is eventually stored as bodyfat. So for anyone looking to burn fat and lose weight, drinking a sugar-laden energy drink to try and achieve this is a pretty stupid move.

Along with bags of caffeine, these drinks also contain all sorts of other unnatural ingredients you've probably never heard of before. I bought three cans of big name brand energy drinks to draw a comparison and I was shocked by the huge number of flavourings, colourings, and other questionable additives in them. Sure, there were some vitamins and natural ingredients included, but these are negligible in my opinion, given that excess sugar robs the body of vitamins and minerals anyway.

Here's how those drinks stacked up:

Brand A

Sugar - 55g (13 teaspoons) per 500ml can.

Ingredients - 20.

Brand B

Sugar - 69g (17 teaspoons) per 500ml can.

Ingredients - 14.

Brand C

Sugar - 39g (9 teaspoons) per 355ml can.

Ingredients - 15.

These cans went straight into the bin after I checked them out and made the comparison for the purposes of this chapter. Below are five strong reasons I'd recommend you do the same.

5 Reasons For Ditching Energy Drinks

#1 The caffeine content can be dangerously high

Caffeine increases alertness and provides a boost in energy but too high doses – while mixed with other ingredients and/or alcohol – can potentially be lethal. Several deaths around the world have been linked to various energy drinks. I won't single out any particular brands because lawsuits are still ongoing in some cases, but if you've been consuming energy drinks it's worth doing some research online before you gulp another drop. You might be shocked at what you discover.

#2 Way too much sugar

One word for the amount of added sugar in the energy drinks cans I've mentioned - ridiculous! Just imagine dropping 17 teaspoons of sugar into a pint glass of water and then drinking it. That's basically what people are doing when they consume this stuff.

Refined sugar in all its man-made forms (including the likes of 'high fructose corn syrup', 'sucrose', 'glucose syrup' etc) is the enemy to good health. Over consumption of sugar is strongly linked to all the big major diseases including cancer, heart disease and diabetes.

#3 They are NOT the same as sports drinks designed for performance enhancement

Sports drinks contain water, smaller amounts of sugar and minerals such as potassium and sodium that are lost during intense physical activity. Many top brands are used to good effect by athletes as they enhance hydration and provide carbohydrates for energy - but don't have the same massive amounts of sugar or stimulating effects as high caffeine energy drinks.

#4 There could be long-term effects medical experts are not aware of yet

The energy drinks market has exploded in recent years and there's little research available on the long term effects of consuming these products regularly.

On the websitesharecare.com, Dr Michael Breus PhD warns that we're still in the early stages of learning about "the full range of effects of energy drinks on physical and mental health, as well as sleep."

#5 There are safer, healthier alternatives

There are a variety of natural foods, drinks and supplements that you can take that can give you an energy boost pre-workout. One unexpected source of energy that is growing in popularity among athletes, particularly endurance runners, is beetroot juice.

It's believed that beetroot juice increases blood and oxygen flow in the body. That's undoubtedly why athletes were using it at the London 2012 Olympics and why US marathon runner Ryan Hall always downs a glass to improve his run time.

I gave it a try last month...and it was too gaggingly disgusting to try again. I share an easier, tastier, simpler pre-workout drink option with you in Part Four which is like rocket fuel for your exercise sessions.

Keeping Your Calories In Check

Calories are important when it comes to fat loss, but do you really want to count how many are in your meals every day? No, me neither.

Life's too short to be doing sums in your head every time you take a bite to eat or have a drink. Fortunately, you don't have to because there's an awesome app worth using to help you keep your calories in check and to optimise your daily nutrition.

I'll come to that soon, but first let's talk about calories and their effect on your weight levels. A calorie, also known as a kilocalorie, is the measure of energy within the food and drink we consume. It provides us with fuel for our daily activities...including those tough weights and sprint sessions I was talking about earlier.

If we regularly take in more calories than we use up every day then naturally we'll gain weight. The reverse is true: to lose weight we must be in a caloric deficit. How many calories we burn each day depends on various factors including age, genetics, sex, and how active you are. A postman out and about delivering mail for hours each day is going to burn more calories than an office worker sitting at their desk all day.

For me personally, I naturally have a high metabolism and exercise 3-4 days per week, meaning that I must take in more calories particularly on workout days to ensure I don't lose weight.

If you're overweight and want to shed bodyfat, it's a must that you cut back on calories until you hit your target. Then you can make adjustments once you've achieved your aim.

There are a couple of ways to figure how many calories an active person generally needs each day. The first is this simple equation which provides an approximate number:

* **Weight loss: bodyweight in pounds x 12 = number of daily calories.**

* **Weight maintenance: bodyweight in pounds x 15 = number of daily calories.**

* **Weight gain: bodyweight in pounds x 18 = number of daily calories.**

This is a formula that gives you a very rough idea, but our bodies are all different and remember there are various other factors which contribute to your caloric needs.

That's where the MyFitnessPal app comes in. It's an amazing tool for not only figuring out an accurate picture of your calorie requirements based on your specific fitness goals, it also helps you keep on top of your nutrition overall easily.

Rather than counting calories, grams of protein, carbs or how much fat is in your foods, you can simply scan barcodes on packaging with the MyFitnessPal app or type in the name of foods and it automatically works it all out for you. Your nutritional stats are easily saved into a daily food diary and you can take full charge of your nutrition in just a few minutes per day.

I use this app with online personal training clients, as do many other health and fitness professionals around the world. While it's not a necessity for you to track your calories or use a food diary in the long term, it's a key tool to use until you burn fat and lose enough weight to hit your fitness target.

If you're looking to burn fat fast and have struggled to lose weight for a while, a perfect combination would be: intermittent fasting + weight training three days per week + a daily caloric deficit. Throw a single 15 minute sprints session per week into the mix and you'll inevitably smash your goal.

To use the MyFitnessPal app you'll have to set up a free account. After that it's fairly easy to use but there are several features you might want to explore, such as saving meal recipes. You can learn how to use the app properly via this YouTube demo video: https://www.youtube.com/watch?v=fu9RKqlmD1Q&t=179s

Delay Your Post-Workout Shake

Have you been told to guzzle a protein shake straight after your workout for maximum muscle, minimal fat?

It's common sense advice. Gulp down a shake filled with the right amount of protein and carbs to flood your system with nutrients. Then the body can get to work on developing muscle and sculpting that awesome new physique you're aiming for.

I did that for the best part of 10 years. Dropping the dumbbell for the last rep of my workout in the gym, grabbing my shaker (already with protein powder inside), and running to fill it up with water so I could have my shake immediately.

The body is in a catabolic (muscle tissue breakdown) state after an intense workout and that flips to anabolic (muscle building) when you provide it with the right nutrients for repair and development.

My thinking process was: the sooner that healthy protein shake hits my stomach the better my body transformation will be. After busting my balls in a heavy weights session, I want to make sure I capitalise on all my hard work.

A while ago that approach has changed - slightly - thanks to the wisdom of the sports nutrition mastermind Ori Hofmekler. (I referred to Ori's work in Part One). In a fascinating interview with American fitness guru Dr Chad Waterbury, Ori Hofmekler revealed that delaying your post-workout shake/meal by 30-60 mins after your training session you can maximise fat burning.

Ori said: "Exercise only initiates the first phase of fat breakdown; it does not grant the completion of the fat-burning process. After exercise there's a substantial increase in the level of circulating free fatty acids coming from adipose tissue, and unless these are mobilized to the liver and muscle for final utilization, most of them will be re-esterfied into triglycerides and re-deposited back in the fat tissues.

"Yes, all your hard work to burn fat will be wasted! In order to grant an effective completion of the fat-burning process you must manipulate your muscle to suck in the circulating free fatty acids that were released by exercise.

"And the way to do that is to wait for 30-60 minutes after exercise before having your recovery meal."

There you have it - exercise is only half of the fat burning process. By delaying your post-workout shake/meal by 30 minutes to one hour this prevents fatty acids from being drawn back into fat tissues; thereby maximising your fat loss efforts.

The interview with Ori, titled 'The Truth About Post Workout Nutrition', is a detailed and very interesting read. Well worth checking out and you can do so by visiting:http://chadwaterbury.com/the-truth-about-post-workout-nutrition/

One Positive Habit Per Week

Meet Steven. A 30-year-old construction worker who has just started dating a girl for the first time since has last relationship ended four years ago.

He's been piling on the pounds for years, not really bothering much about it, but suddenly decides now is the time to sort out his health and fitness (again). He wants to improve his appearance, be more confident…thinking it'll help him hang onto his new girlfriend.

Steven's biggest issue - his diet. He boozes every Friday and Saturday (sometimes the odd weeknight too), he rarely sleeps well as a result, he eats takeaways 3-4 days per week, dinner is usually followed by 4 or 5 biscuits, he drinks a two litre bottle of Coke while at work, and the only time he sees vegetables are when he walks past them in the supermarket while heading straight for the pizzas.

Not exactly the healthiest of lifestyles and Steven knows it. There's plenty to change and he's determined to do it because he wants to drop two stones, maybe even three if possible.

So, the diet begins. No to booze, no to biscuits, no to pizza, no to the takeaway meals. He's gone cold turkey on the junk. And it's yes to low fat yoghurts, tasteless 'healthy' microwave meals, and generally starving himself to try and get rid of the flab.

Fast forward three weeks: he's lost barely 3lbs, is miserable, been arguing with his girlfriend as a result…and is so pissed off with it all that he's just ordered a large Big Mac Meal, two double cheeseburgers, a strawberry milkshake, and a donut at McDonald's.

True story. Although his name's not actually Steven - and I think he ordered 10 chicken nuggets and an apple pie aswell. Here's the moral of the story: if you try to change everything at once it'll likely end up in failure.

There's quite a lot to take in from this book, training and nutrition wise, especially if you've not done much exercise until now or didn't really have a clue about following a healthy diet.

This can mean an entire lifestyle change and wrestling with a lot of bad old habits. These are like programmes we've created over years…and it's not a straightforward 'deprogramming' process simply because you've read this book.

I'll put it this way: if you try to implement everything at once you'll likely fuck things up. And I don't want you to fuck things up.

These exercise and nutritional strategies already covered in this book have long been proven for blitzing bodyfat and helping people get in much better shape. But it's wise to introduce these positive changes - and remove the negative ones - *gradually* in order for you to be successful.

Otherwise you'll likely end up feeling overwhelmed and it'll create resistance within you to keep pushing on. So what should you do?

When it comes to exercise focus on one thing at a time - and then build upon it.

When it comes to your nutrition make one change at a time - and then build upon this too.

When I take on new personal training clients, I ask them to fill in a short questionnaire about their diet and nutrition so I can get a clear picture of their eating habits and to see what we can improve.

In most cases, there are numerous foods and drinks they should be cutting back on in order to see the changes they want. There are often many healthy foods they should be including more of.

They're desperate to hear about all of these to help them hit their health and fitness goals sooner. But it won't do any good bombarding them with everything at once. It leads to information overload, trying to make too many changes at once, and effectively moving onto to a restrictive 'diet'. I don't do diets. Instead, we make gradual changes by introducing **one positive habit per week**.

Where should you start? What should be implemented in what order? I think it's important to put core practices in place first; the ones that will get quickest results. Then you can keep adding in one new positive habit per week.

For example, if you currently go out jogging twice per week to try and burn fat then I'd swap that for three weight training sessions at the gym. This is a core foundational change to your exercise regime.

The following week you could focus on your diet and get started with intermittent fasting. Again, this is probably the best place to start when it comes to diet and nutrition. Stay focused only on skipping breakfast for that week, with no other diet distractions.

By week two, you've proven you can stick with intermittent fasting and now it's time to build upon that. You realise your high sugar intake is one of the main reasons for being overweight, so you resolve to only have dessert after your dinner one day this week instead of 5-6 days per week. This is your target for week two, don't worry about fixing anything else in your diet for now.

By week three you're not only gaining momentum, but you're gaining confidence and strengthening your willpower because you've achieved your goals so far. This week's positive habit to add to the previous two - cook double the amount of food for dinner this week and take the other serving into work the next day. Your freshly cooked food is a much better option to the junk food you've been buying in the work canteen or from the fast food joint down the road.

You see where I'm going with this? It's easy to understand, easy to implement and, most importantly, it's much easier to maintain. Don't worry, if you have the odd slip-up. We all do, and again it's because we're so used to our old negative habits even if they're not good for our health.

The key is to stay focused on one positive habit per week and do your best to achieve it each day. Keep stacking those habits, keep building your confidence, and watch as your burn fat faster than you've ever done before.

Part Four

Fat Burning Hacks

Training In The Morning On An Empty Stomach

Remember being told that breakfast is the "most important meal of the day"?

Maybe for kids going to school to help them focus on their education without their bellies grumbling. For adults? The health benefits of skipping breakfast extend way beyond burning fat and staying lean, but actually include improved digestion, detoxification, cell regeneration, the list goes on.

After doing plenty of research into why intermittent fasting was good for me, I was more than content to give brekkie a break. But no food in my stomach before my workouts? **I'm not advising this for lifting heavy weights**, but when it comes to an early morning sprints session an empty belly is the only way to go.

It was only after I began early morning sprint training sessions with my mate Ryan that I began experimenting with exercising on an empty stomach. We got up at 7am to get ready for sprints and I quickly wolfed down a bowl of porridge, thinking I'd really need those carbs to get me through the tough high intensity session. Ryan, as usual, decided to have his breakfast later in the morning and did his sprints on an empty stomach.

Here's what happened: by the third sprint I was close to spewing, the food felt like a heavy weight in my stomach, and I developed an instant headache. Next time around, I sprinted on an empty stomach and, despite worrying I'd be dizzy because there was no food fuel in my body, I performed much better.

Guess what else I noticed a few weeks down the line? The thin layer of flab around my belly had disappeared and my abs were properly on show again. As described earlier, sprint training has a huge fat burning effect, but combining this with training in the morning on an empty stomach moved things up a gear.

American doctor and health guru, Joseph Mercola, is a big proponent of exercising early in the morning on an empty stomach. For people aiming to burn fat, he says that working out in the AM while still in a fasted state following sleeping is a wise move.

He explains that the combination of fasting and exercising maximises the impact of cellular factors and catalysts, which result in the breakdown of fat for energy. Training on an empty stomach effectively forces your body to burn up fat.

Here's another reason to drag yourself out of bed and exercise in the AM…you're much more likely to stick to your weekly training regime. When you training in the morning you can't make the excuse that you ran out of time, or that a meeting came up, or that you had to work late at the office. If training is your start to the day, then it's less likely to be ditched for something else.

An Energy Booster

When I say training on an empty stomach, I'm not being *completely* honest. I've usually given myself a cheeky wee boost. It's something you might drink every day, something you might love the smell of, and something that'll not only supercharge your training but boost fat burning by around 10%.

Your cup is served in the next chapter.

Supercharge Your Workouts With Black Coffee

If you're worried that you'll struggle to get through a tough workout in the morning on an empty stomach, then relax and pour yourself a cuppa.

A black coffee will give your bags of beans in the gym. The caffeine will flow through your system and provide more energy than any bowl of cereal. Best of all: it's been proven to take stoke your fat burning fire.

The caffeine in coffee not only provides the fuel you need for training, but it can cause fatty acids to be used for energy rather than glycogen. Studies have shown that coffee also speeds up metabolism and fat oxidation, which means more fat is burned throughout the day.

I'm guessing there are one of two thoughts going through your mind right now…

"Can it *really* be that effective at burning fat?" or "…I fucking HATE coffee!"

I've lost count of the amount of people who've told me they can't drink the stuff. That it makes them feel sick. That they'd rather drink a shot of their own piss. (Well, maybe not the last statement).

I'll be honest, I was never really a big fan of coffee. In fact, I'm still not…but I neck a cup of it anyway because of the awesome effect it has on my training. One cup of black coffee (yes, no sugar or cream) and made from ground coffee beans rather than instant granules that have been ridiculously processed and robbed the coffee of its natural antioxidants.

Yes, coffee actually contains antioxidants that can clear out toxins in the body, supposedly slow ageing, and apparently reduce the risk of cancer. To enjoy these benefits make your coffee using organic beans or freshly ground coffee, rather than the instant garbage. And go easy on it as health experts recommend no more than 400mg of caffeine (roughly three mugs of coffee) per day.

7 Reasons Why Having A Black Coffee Pre-Workout Is A Hot Idea

1. Performance boost

Coffee can be the difference between shaving a few seconds off your running time or adding a couple more exercises to your training regime.

This was proven back in 1992 when a group of athletes were given 3g of coffee before a 1500m treadmill run. The study, published in the British Journal of Sports Medicine showed that those who drank the coffee finished their run 4.2 secs faster on average than the control group.

2. Increased energy

The caffeine in coffee can provide a much-needed charge to your batteries before exercise. Just don't go nuts as excessive caffeine intake has been shown to have side effects such as increased heart rate and insomnia.

Remember, medics widely recommend that no more than 400mg of caffeine (three mugs) is consumed per day, while the limit is 200mg for pregnant women.

3. More fat is burned

Some health experts say that coffee can increase your basal metabolic rate by around 10%, while others say as much as 20%. I expect the figure varies from person to person, but what's not in question is that coffee can speed up your metabolism.

This means more calories burned and more fat melted away.

4. Improved focus

Along with more energy to burn during exercise, black coffee also keeps you alert and provides an increase in mental focus. This helps you stick with it and get the most out of each workout.

5. Can help the unfit become more active

A group of sedentary men hopped on exercise bikes after drinking caffeine for a study in 2012. Researchers were so impressed by the performance of these unfit guys that they reckon the boost given by caffeine could "motivate sedentary men to participate in exercise more often and so reduce adverse effects of inactivity on health."

6. Reduced muscle soreness

Drinking coffee before exercise can reduce muscle soreness post-workout by up to 48%, according to the following study published in the March 2007 issue of Journal Of Pain.

7. It's a healthy alternative to energy drinks

The popularity of energy drinks has exploded to the point that it is now a multi-billion dollar industry. As mentioned earlier, health experts have repeatedly warned about the dangers of these drinks due to the mixture of high levels of caffeine, sugar and various other ingredients.

Best steering clear when there's a healthier, safer alternative. Now you have seven good reasons to drink coffee. Serve up one mug – without the cream and sugar – 30-60 mins before you next exercise to stir up those energy levels.

Give Green Tea The Green Light

Are you a tea with two sugars and milk kinda person? Do you have 3,4,5 cups per day...maybe 17 when you're hungover or feeling like shit?

Why not ditch at least some of those cups for **green tea** instead to give your body a fat-burning boost? I'm drinking my second cup of the day (in my special Kylie Minogue mug) as I type this.

If you want to give your body a helping hand to slim down the waistline and lose any jiggly bits, then it's time to give green tea the green light. Scientific studies have shown that there's something quite special going on with those green tea leaves and its fat burning magic is becoming well known.

Green contains catechins which naturally raise levels of the key fat burning hormone norepinephrine. Norepinephrine elevates metabolism levels and increases the rate of fatty acid utilisation...meaning that your cuppa green can turn you into a blubber burning boss!

What Brand And How Many Cups?

This is where you'll have to do a bit of research because the quality of tea leaves and catechin content can vary dramatically. This is all down to where the tea plant is grown, if it's classed as organic or not, and how it's actually processed. Studies have shown that even the brew time and water temperature can affect the amount of catechins in the cuppa.

If you're looking for a top quality brew than Green Tea Lovers (greentealovers.com) is a good place to start. The New York based company sources high quality, organic, Fair Trade green tea from around the world and boasts that its teas have "ultra high antioxidant levels". Otherwise, if you choose to buy at your local supermarket then it's worth paying a little more for a better quality brand, looking out for organic tea bags.

Green tea reaches its fat-burning potential with around 400-500 milligrams of ECGC—the most active catechin—per day. That's around four cups of strongly brewed tea.

A simple alternative is to opt for a green tea extract (GTE) supplement. GTE pills are becoming more widely used by people looking to cut their bodyfat levels. They are sold cheaply on leading sports supplements websites such as MyProtein.com and allow you to take green tea in a more concentrated form and fully benefit from the fat burning effects of green tea. These tablets are natural, safe, and effective for weight loss, backed up by many customer reviews online.

Remember to check the labels and not to exceed the recommended dosage because GTE also contains caffeine.

The Magic Of Lemon Water

This last chapter will finish oh so beautifully with one of the first things I do every morning. I repeated it and repeated it constantly until it became a habit just like brushing my teeth. Now it's second nature and undoubtedly one of the best things I do for my health.

One pint glass.

Filled with lukewarm water.

And the juice of half a lemon.

So easy to do. Also so easy not to do when you're scrambling around late for work or getting the kids ready for school. But if you make a conscious effort to have this refreshing drink for at least a month you'll discover it's an amazing start to each day. It can also boost your fat-burning efforts because lemon juice contains pectin fibre which helps reduce your appetite.

There are plenty other health benefits you can experience simply by buying in 3 or 4 lemons per week and adding the juice to water every morning. One of the first, and most obvious, reasons for doing this is that we're typically most dehydrated when we first wake up. The combination of taking in no fluids while we're snoozing, combined with sweating during our sleep, results in dehydration.

Of course, the tell-tale sign that you need some h2o in your system is if your pee is coloured and not clear. This is usually the situation in the morning. This is your cue to head to kitchen, heat a pint of water a little, pour into a pint glass, and then squeeze the juice of half a lemon before drinking.

Not only does it taste awesome, there are many reasons for enjoying a glass of lemon water. Below are just some of the main ones.

9 Benefits Of Drinking Lemon Water

#1 Better digestion

Lemon juice has antibacterial qualities and helps rid the intestines of toxins. Too much processed food in the typical Western diet often leads to digestive issues, such as constipation and heartburn for many people. These are clear signs that your body's struggling to break down what you've been consuming and this can lead to toxins floating around in your system.

The antibacterial effect of lemon juice helps flush toxins and bacteria, which is important at the start of your day before you continue eating more food.

#2 Immune system boost

Lemons and other citrus fruits contain high amounts of vitamin C, which is one of the most important antioxidant vitamins for boosting the immune system. Vitamin C helps protect cells from damaging free radicals, is needed for healing wounds, and contributes to maintaining strong bones and teeth.

#3 It contains other vitamins and minerals

While not on the same scale as vitamin C, lemon juice also contains the B vitamins riboflavin, folate, thiamin and B6. These are important for metabolism, helping the body convert carbohydrates, proteins and fats into glucose to be used for energy. A deficiency in B vitamins leads to tiredness and fatigue.

Lemon juice also contains the minerals magnesium, calcium and is particularly high in potassium, which is good for heart health and the function of your brain and nervous system.

#4 Cancer protection

Compounds called limonoids are found in lemons. These also have antioxidant properties, helping to destroy free radicals in the body. Limonoids also have the ability to help prevent the development and growth of cancer cells, according to a report in the April 2005 issue of the Journal of Nutrition. Tested against human cancer cells, limonoids not only halted their growth but were also responsible for the death of the cancer cells.

#5 Clearer skin

The antioxidants in lemon juice help to decrease blemishes on your skin. As it's detoxifying to your blood, it helps maintain a healthy complexion.

#7 Blood sugar regulation

Another compound found in lemons called hesperidin can have a positive impact on the function of enzymes in the body that affect blood sugar levels. As this can help lower blood sugar levels, the result is that this compound can protect the body from the development of diabetes. This was concluded in the January 2010 issue of the Journal of Clinical Biochemistry and Nutrition, which also reported that hesperidin has cholesterol-lowering effects too.

#8 Helps prevent kidney stones

Kidney stones are solid mineral formations that can build up in the kidneys. The citric acid found in lemons is just what the doctor ordered for preventing kidney stones. Health experts report that more citrate in your system can halt the formation of calcium stones. Lemons and limes have the most citric acid, while oranges, grapefruits and berries also contain large amounts.

#9 Helps fight viral infections

Again this is down to the antibacterial qualities of lemons. In studies it has been shown to kill deadly diseases such as malaria, cholera, diptheria, and typhoid. Squeeze the life out of pathogens with some fresh lemon water.

Want to kickstart a leaner, healthier lifestyle and do what you can to protect yourself from various illnesses? A simple pint of lemon water every day could go a long way to helping you achieve this.

Conclusion

In four parts, 21 chapters, and nearly 17,000 words we've gone over a wide variety of *physical* actions you can take to Burn Fat Fast.

Changes to your meal timing, what's included in your meals, and what you should avoid like the plague. We've looked at your weekly training regime, why weight training is much more effective at burning fat than cardio and why intense sprint training is the secret to a leaner, stronger body.

You can now make some tweaks that'll contribute to your body sculpting mission such as delaying your post-workout meal and building upon one positive habit per week.

You're now armed to go to war on your bodyfat with fat burning hacks that are not only easy to implement, but have been proven to deliver results time and again.

I've saved the biggest hack of all until now…

One that is the superglue for holding everything else together and making sure it doesn't break.

I'm talking about hacking your **mindset** and forcing a complete shift from your usual pattern of thinking when it comes to your health and fitness - and your self image.

All of the strategies I've described up until now work well for burning fat, improving your fitness levels and getting in great shape. I have zero doubt that if you implement these exercise and dietary principles as described that you'll achieve your particular goal; whether that's getting rid of some stubborn belly fat or losing a considerable amount of weight.

Forget how many times you may have failed in the past, this is a new start and you now have highly effective strategies that have spawned countless success stories. Best of all: the approach in this book doesn't involve any crazy yo-yo dieting or extreme exercise routine you cannot maintain.

It's do-able, manageable, and sustainable in the long term. You can achieve great results - but I want you to **maintain them**. That's why we must conclude by focusing on mindset right now.

This was the big issue for a recent personal training client of mine called Johnny. He'd been working with another PT for months, wasn't happy with his rate of progress, and decided to quit.

 A couple of months later, pissed off with the weight piling on and with another gust of willpower, he asked to join my 10 week training and nutrition coaching programme. He was two stones overweight but after looking closely at his diet, it wasn't exactly the worst.

We changed up his gym routine to focus on heavy weight training with compound exercises and he was already damn good at many of these moves. In fact, he was a boss at squats and deadlifts and was soon lifting more than me.

After a couple of weeks it became apparent what was really holding Johnny back…his mindset and doubts about what he was capable of.

He told me: "When I tried to lose weight the last time around I got rid of just a few pounds but that was it. Every time I stepped on the scales I knew it would be the same. I kept thinking, 'is this a waste of time?', 'am I doing the exercises wrong?'

"I stepped up my training to six days per week and then ended up even more pissed off because I wasn't getting the results for the amount of effort I was putting in.

"I'm always willing to work hard but it always seems like I'm so far away from getting anywhere."

The more he spoke the clearer our #1 problem became: Johnny was already defeated before he began.

Have you ever stopped to properly listen to your thoughts as you work your ass off to become healthier and fitter? That nagging, annoying, relentless inner critic whispering words of doubt in your head, even when you're clearly working hard towards your goal.

"I still can't see any changes in my body, feels like I'm getting nowhere…"

"Maybe I'm just not working hard enough, maybe I'm just doing it all wrong…"

"Am I wasting my time at the gym?"

"My diet hasn't been great the past couple of days, who am I kidding I can lose this weight?"

Who needs enemies when you've got the harshest critic around inside your own head? I don't care who you are or what weight, age, or nationality you are, we all have insecurities and body image issues to some degree. But there are two very important steps you must take to develop the right mindset for achieving your goals.

#1 Stand guard over your mind.

Don't let your inner critic take over. He'll take full charge and fuck everything up. When those doubts, negative thoughts and criticisms start creeping in, bat them right out of the park.

This may take a firm conscious effort for a while because many of us have become masters at beating ourselves up. Instead, keep praising yourself for the positive action steps you're taking every day to become a healthier, stronger, better version of yourself.

#2 Act like you've <u>already achieved</u> what you're aiming for.

If you're always thinking in terms of "I want this…" or "I want to achieve that…", you're creating a sense of lack. You're simply reinforcing that you're not where you want to be, and it's going to make it all the harder to get there. Instead, behave like you're *already* lean, strong and in the best shape of your life.

The subconscious mind can't tell a white lie from what's real. Keep feeding it this image of you having already achieved your health and fitness goals - while you continue to work hard - and the body will eventually follow suit.

I said at the beginning of this book that burning fat is easy…and I'm sticking to my guns. Intermittent fasting is easy…much easier than trying out 23,056 different diets in your lifetime.

Limiting your sugar intake every day is easy…much easier than developing diabetes, heart disease or some other serious illness.

Keeping an eye on your calories is easy…introducing one positive habit per week is easy…as is ditching energy drinks, downing a pint of lemon water in the morning, and giving green tea a try.

What's not quite so easy is sprint training. In fact, the first time you do it you may even feel like your heart's going to burst through your chest. But it's so ridiculously effective for burning bodyfat that you'd be a fool to not give it a go. One 15 minute session per week is all it takes and, while it's tough as hell, real change only occurs outside of your comfort zone.

As for weight training, I've long argued that this is the most effective form of exercise for men and women looking to develop a strong, lean, toned body. I touched upon the importance of compound exercises, lifting heavy, and why lifting weights just three days per week is all that's required to get in great shape.

I go into much more detail on this in my book 'Strength Training Program 101: Build Muscle & Burn Fat…In Less Than 3 Hours Per Week'. However, you can also download my exercise guide e-book for free by visiting: www.weighttrainingistheway.com/exercise-demos

I hope you've enjoyed reading this book and, if so, I'd be hugely grateful if you left a review on Amazon.

You now have the knowledge and tools to Burn Fat Fast, and transform your overall bodyshape and health.

Work hard. Have faith. Believe in yourself.

About The Author

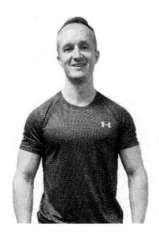

Marc McLean is a 30 something-year-old online personal training and nutrition coach from Loch Lomond in Scotland. He owns Weight Training Is The Way and is a health and fitness writer for leading websites including The Good Men Project, Mind Body Green, and Healthgreatness.com

Marc is also author of the Strength Training 101 book series on Amazon, which includes:

Strength Training Program 101: Build Muscle & Burn Fast…In Less Than 3 Hours Per Week;

Strength Training Nutrition 101: Build Muscle & Burn Fat Easily…A Healthy Way Of Eating You Can Actually Maintain;

Meal Prep Recipe Book: 50 Simple Recipes For Health & Fitness Nuts;

Strength Training For Women: Burn Fat Effectively…And Sculpt The Body You've Always Dreamed Of.

Have any questions about the strategies included in this book, or looking for some strength training or nutritional advice? Feel free to email Marc or reach out to him via social media.

Email: marc@weighttrainingistheway.com

Website: www.weighttrainingistheway.com

Facebook: www.facebook.com/weighttrainingistheway

Instagram: www.instagram.com/weight_training_is_the_way

Printed in Great Britain
by Amazon